How to be a
Winner for Dinner

AUTHORED AND ILLUSTRATED BY

GINA COLAIZZO

DEDICATION

This children's book is dedicated to every science and art teacher that I have had during my life. And if it wasn't for my parents, who made sacrifices to give me the best education from day one, I would not have been taught by these amazing individuals.

Those who have particularly inspired me include Jeff Mordan, Chris Taranta, & Lynn Paige from The Philadelphia School, Mr. Baris & Mrs. Wagner from The Shipley school, and Dr. Reynolds, Jim Tioa, Ed Kerns, Dr. Gabel, Dr. Talarico from Lafayette College

ACKNOWLEDGMENTS

I would like to acknowledge my parents, Dominic & Rachael Colaizzo and the staff and interns at Children's National Medical Center, Robert Keating M.D., Suresh Magge M.D., John Myseros M.D., Amanda Yaun M.D., Nora Taranto, Tyler Amina, Brent Earley-Jones, Tiffani DeFreitas, & Jessica Wisneiwski, for their thoughtful constructive criticism. I would also like to acknowledge Diane Aschenbrenner, MS, RN and Amanda Mazaleski, MSN, RN, ONC, CNL for their support during the beginning of my nursing career.

i

My name is Justin Apple and I live in Delaware.
Being 10 years old, freedom I declare.
Yet dinner in my family is an ordinary act.
Attendance is required, as if I signed a contract.

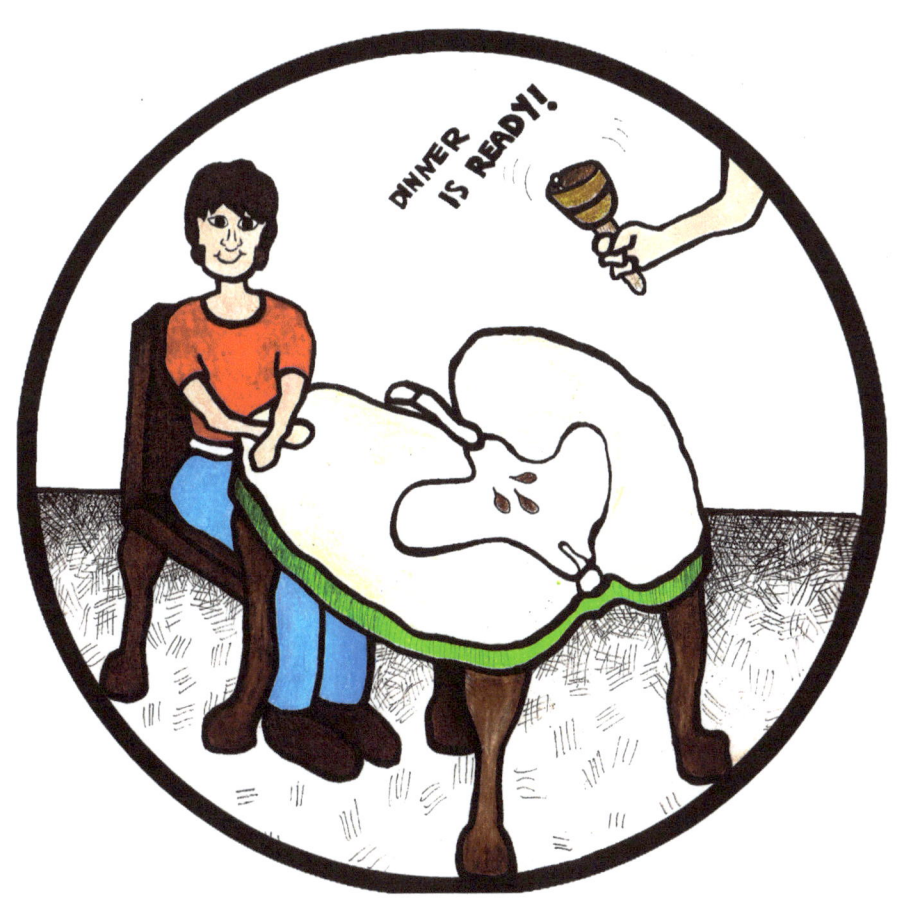

3

Ever since I was a boy, I never ate alone.
My Pappa has a garden, so all our food's homegrown.
He gives his stock to Momma, to see what she'll create
while I quietly wait for dinner, with an empty dinner plate.
There are some days Mom serves us food that I do not care for
in which case I escape down to the corner store.

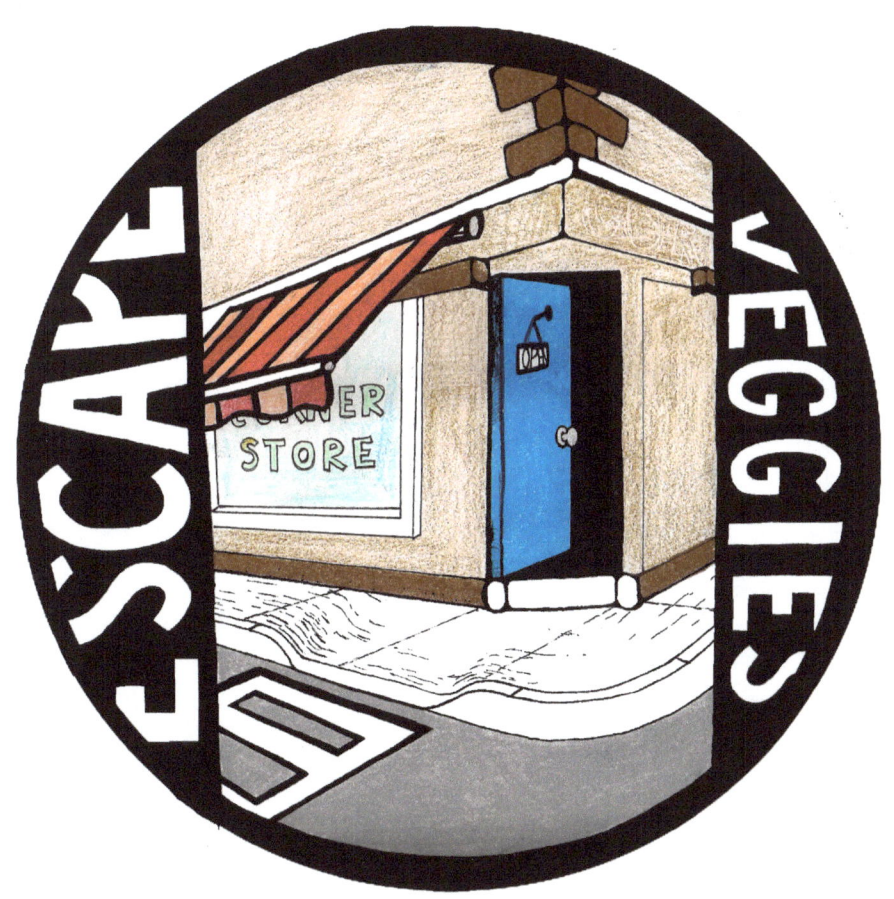

Every night at dinner, she serves at least one veggie,
and when she looks away, I give them all to Reggie.
Reggie is my brother, who eats just like a boar
and gets on Momma's good side by asking for some more.

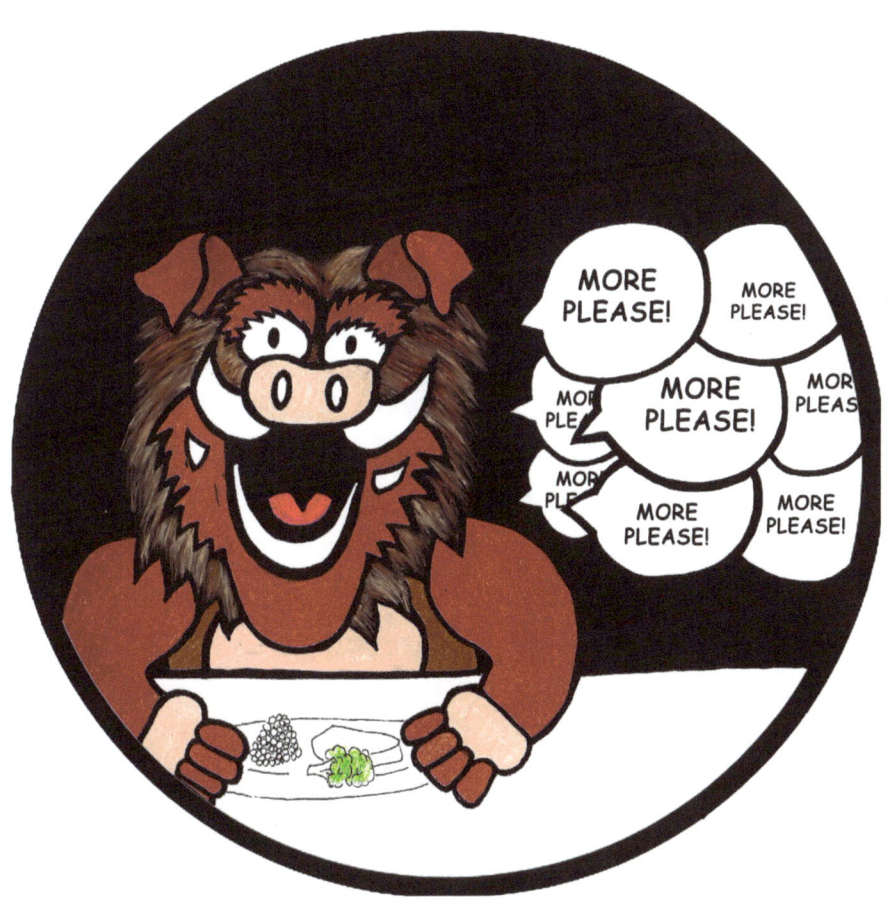

On Monday we eat mushrooms, which daunts me in my sleep,
I think my Momma buys them as they can be pretty cheep.
On Tuesday it's tomatoes, which is technically a fruit.
Mom puts it on my plate, which causes a dispute.
Wednesday winter squash is served, in many shapes and sizes,
which only leaves it much more prone to come with some surprises.
On Thursday we eat turnips, Mom serves it as puree
with the knowledge that its packed with lots of vitamin C.
On Friday we eat fennel, a hearty hollow herb,
when used just as a relish, it's really quite superb.
Sweet potatoes Saturday, she buys them by the sack.
She uses them to make every single kind of snack.
On Sunday we eat snow peas, which we eat in tiny pods,
and if we fail to finish them they form an army squad.
Then Monday rolls around and the cycle starts again,
and Momma only serves us others every now and then.

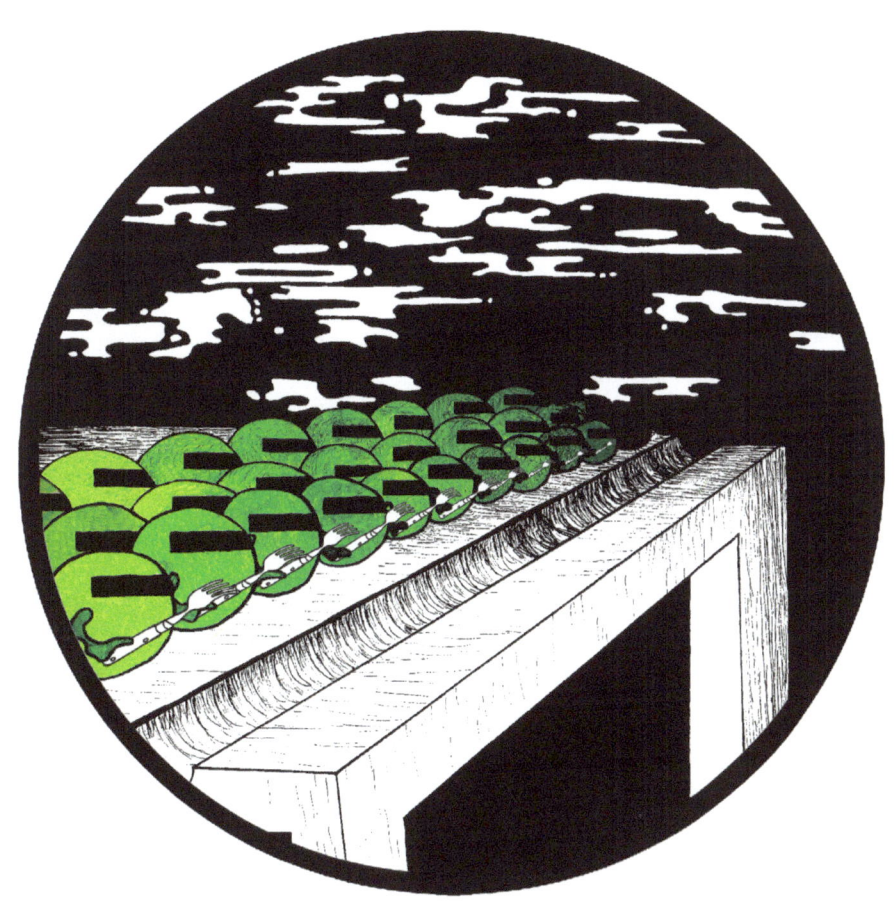

My Poppa seems to like the food my Mom prepares.
He eats them in a joyful state to show my Mom he cares.
Eating veggies everyday makes an active life.
Dad claims that it's the reason, he married his dear wife.
No matter what I do to avoid the night's cuisine,
there is no easy way to avert my Mom's routine.
But just because my family likes them doesn't mean that I have to.
I wonder how they'll taste when they're mixed up in a stew.

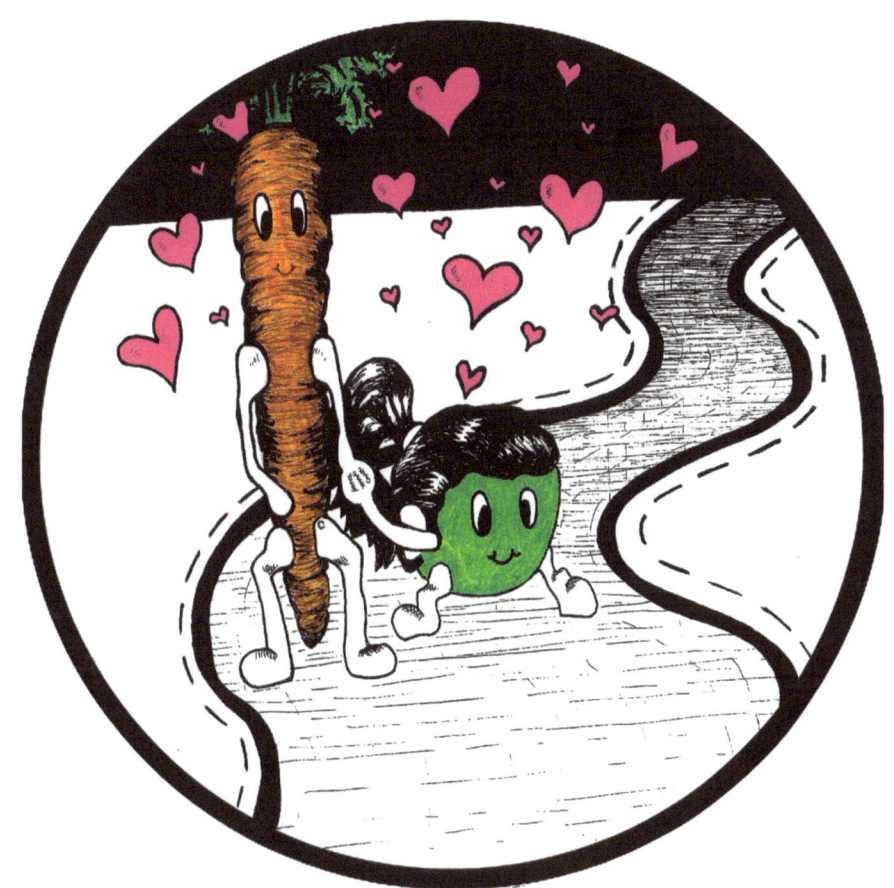

If lucky I will eat the serving on my plate.
I've looked for recipes that will make veggies taste great.
Doctors recommend five total in each day.
They claim the aging process, it's certain to delay.
At the rate my Mom proceeds in only serving one,
I wouldn't be surprised if my aging has begun.
At this rate I am scared, that I will age too fast.
I'll need to eat a ton, to make up for the past.
There has to be a way, for veggies to taste good.
So I can eat my veggies, like any doctor would.

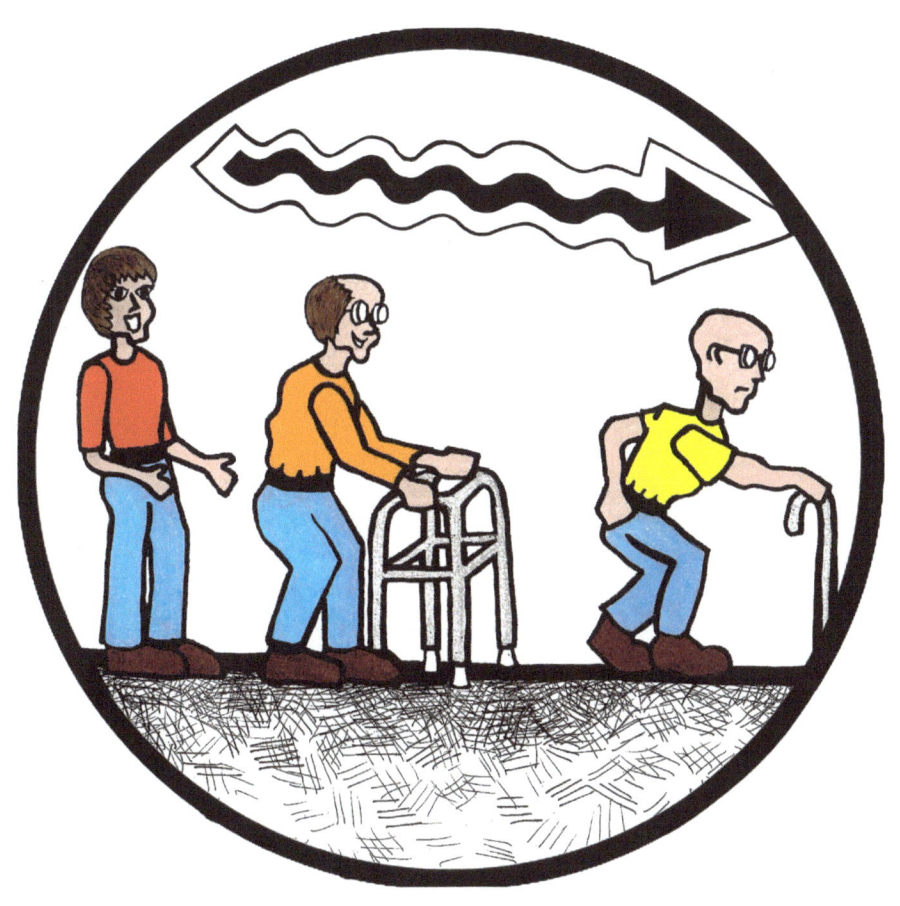

So I went to Baker Bob, with some veggies in my hand,
hoping I could save them, from being way too bland.
He handed me a bucket, crammed with sugar and a spoon
saying "Fill a pot with butter in the early afternoon!"

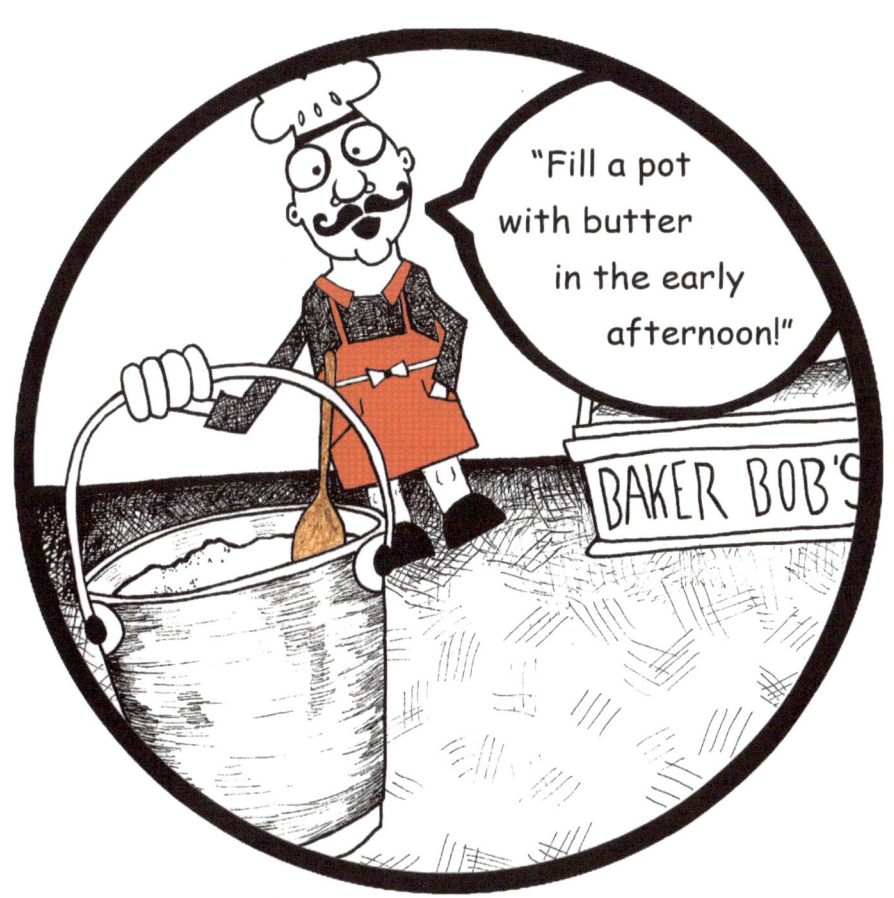

So I took the bucket home, taking his advice,
filled a pot with veggies, and a side of steamed brown rice.

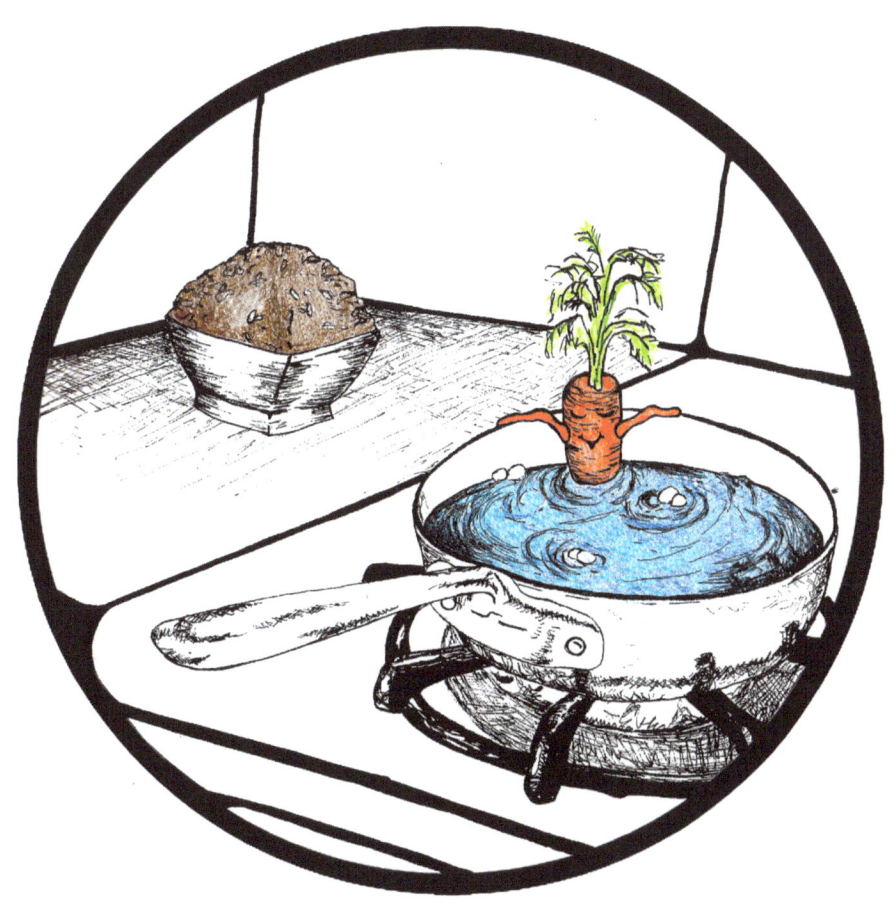

The spoon I used to stir, while I added other stuff,
using my own instinct to gauge when there's enough.
The butter added flavor, as an extra-added gloss,
while the sugar added sweetness for a tasty scrumptious sauce.

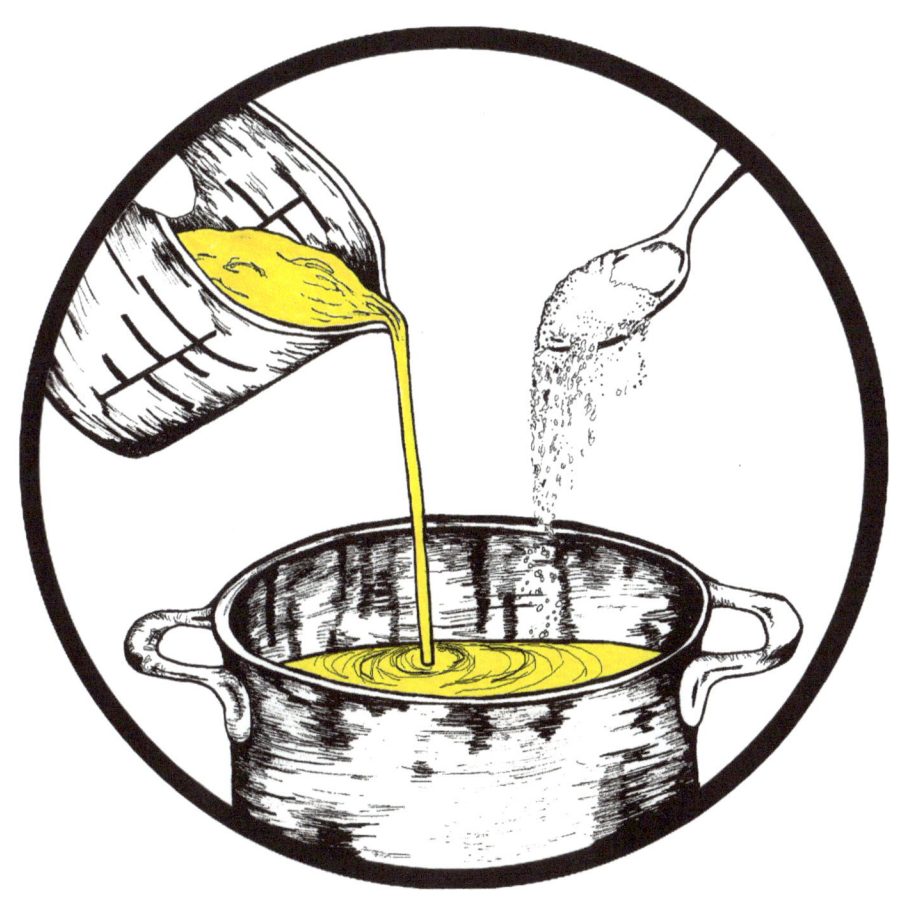

I offered some to Poppa, with some after dinner snacks
to which he kindly said, "there is something that it lacks".
And then he softly stated "it needs pepper and some salt."
I fetched the shakers from the den, and hoped to fix the fault.

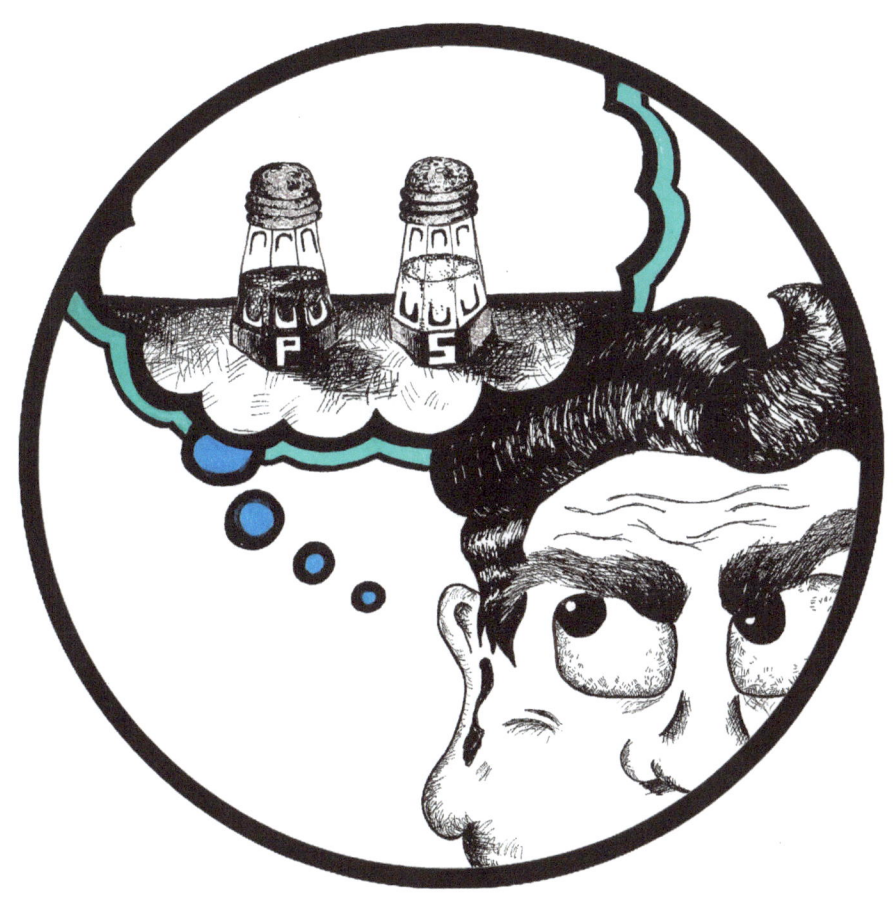

21

A sprinkle here, a sprinkle there, I added to the stew,
and right before my very eyes, it made it taste anew.
I asked my family if they liked it, to which my brother said,
"I swear its even better when you add some extra bread."

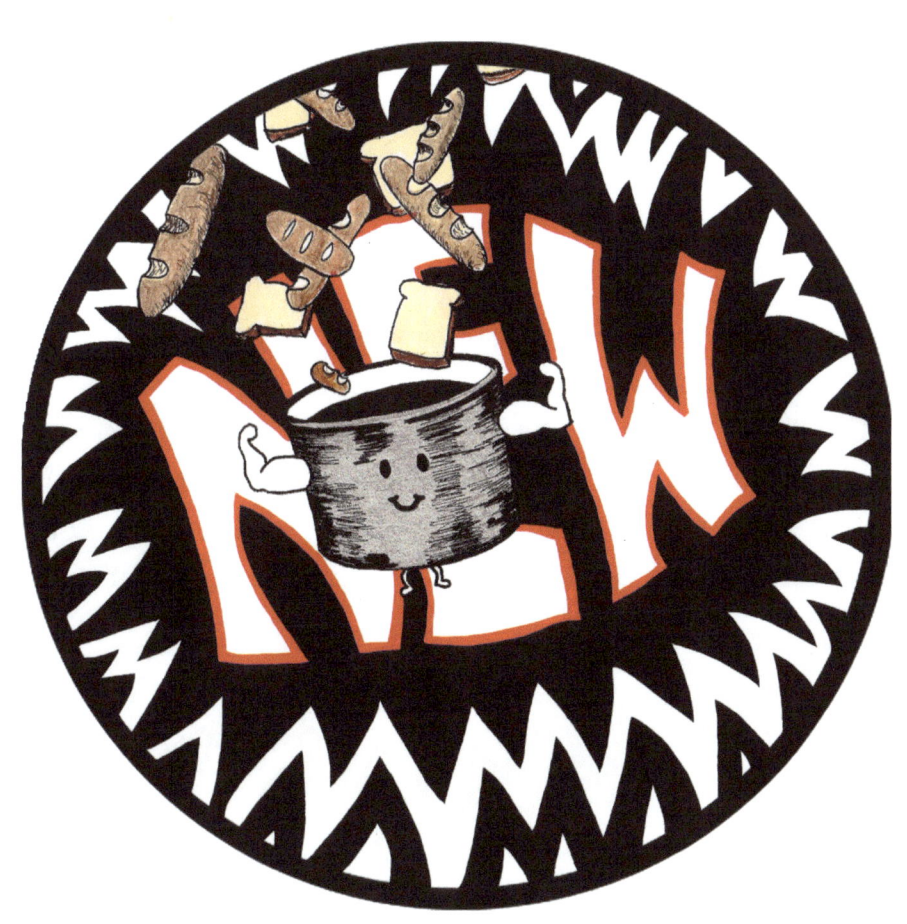

Now at night with dinner, my Mom serves more than one
and eating all those veggies, has come to be quite fun.
The stew has made her able to mix in lots of foods
in which a person eats it and it brightens up their mood.
I eat them in the morning, at lunch and for a snack,
hoping to make up for, all those I used to lack.

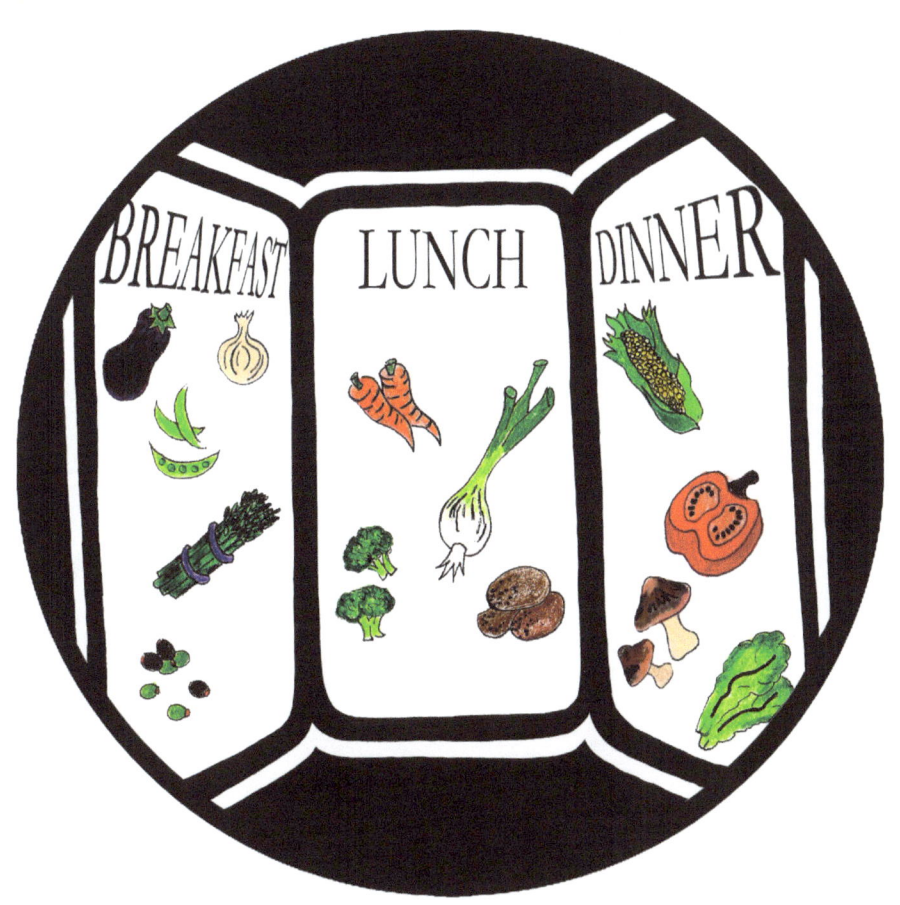

The next appointment at the Docs I told him of the news,
to which he calmly asked, "how much butter do you use?"
I told him just enough to make it taste just like dessert.
He said that if I ate too much it could cause my chest to hurt.
"Butter's filled with fat which is hard to split apart
and clogs up all the pipes that lead into your heart."

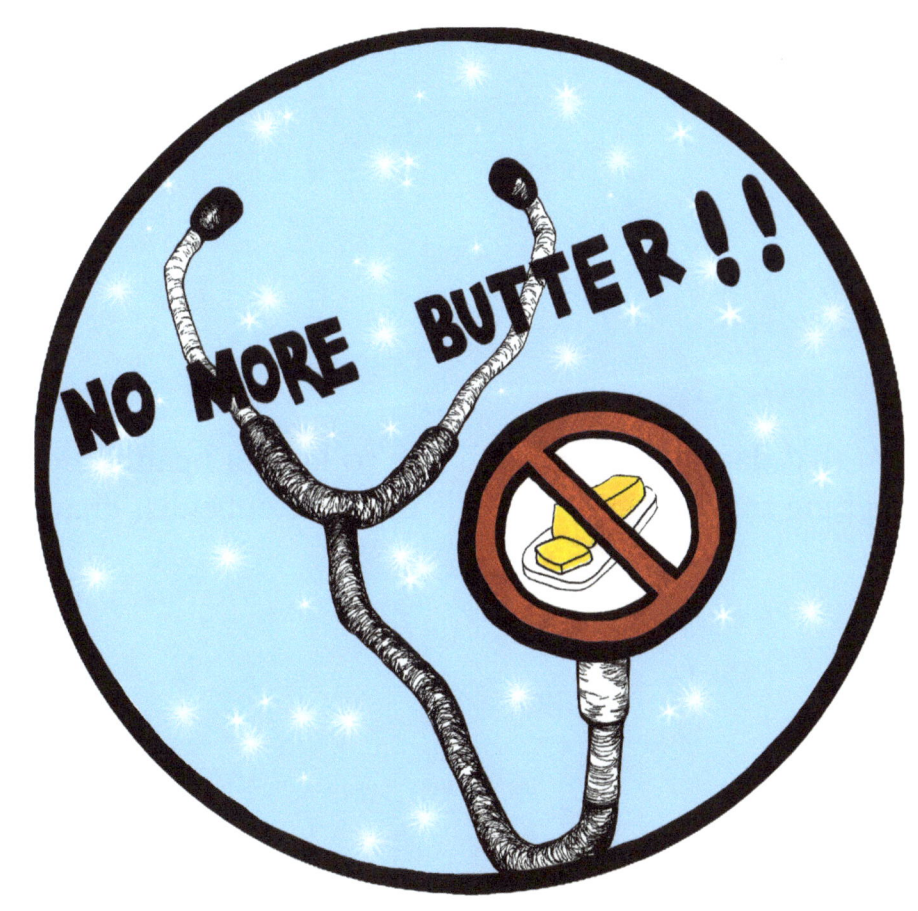

From that day on, I use much less to keep a healthy heart, keeping track of all the foods in a diet checklist chart.

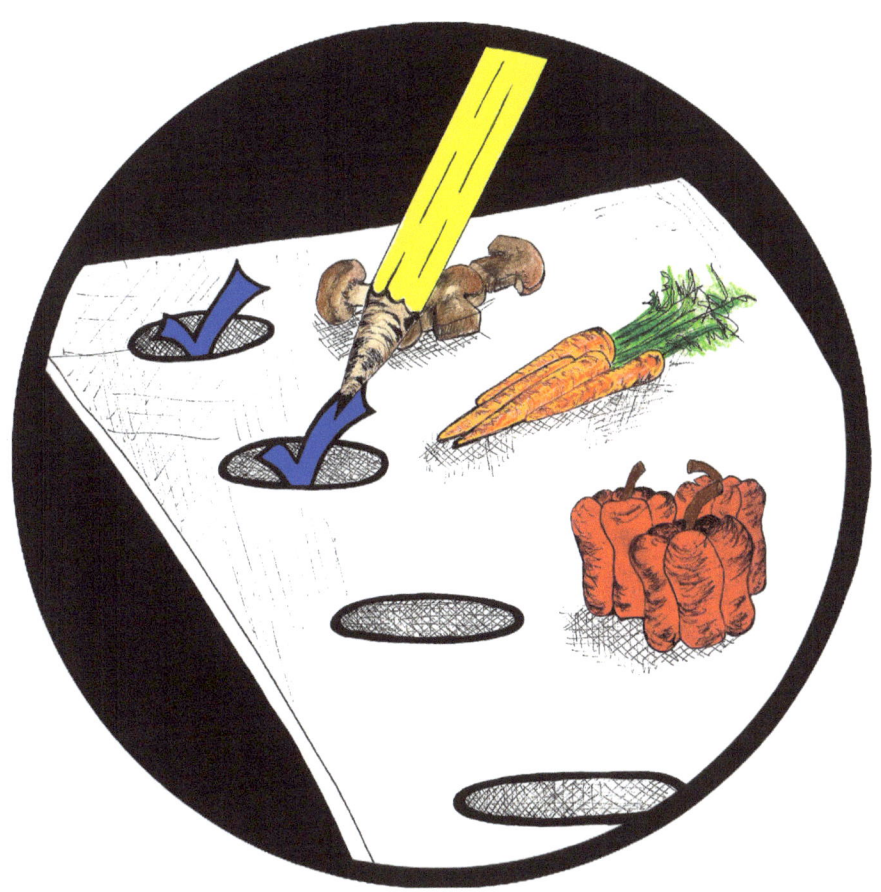

But every now and then, I'll add a spoon or two.
Things in moderation, is something I can do.
I told my Doctor, just to see what he would say,
and his response was "Just don't eat it everyday."

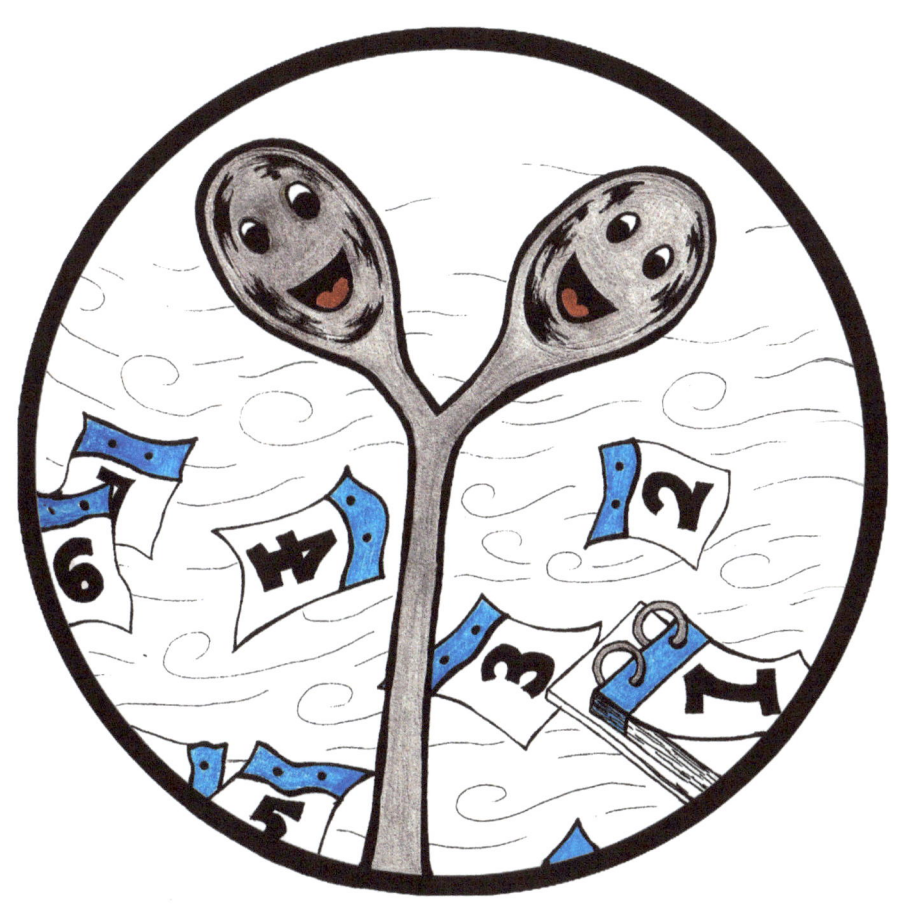

Every night at dinner, I always eat a veggie,
making sure to eat them all before my brother Reggie.
And once a week, as my doctor said I could,
I'll add some salted butter, so that it will taste good.

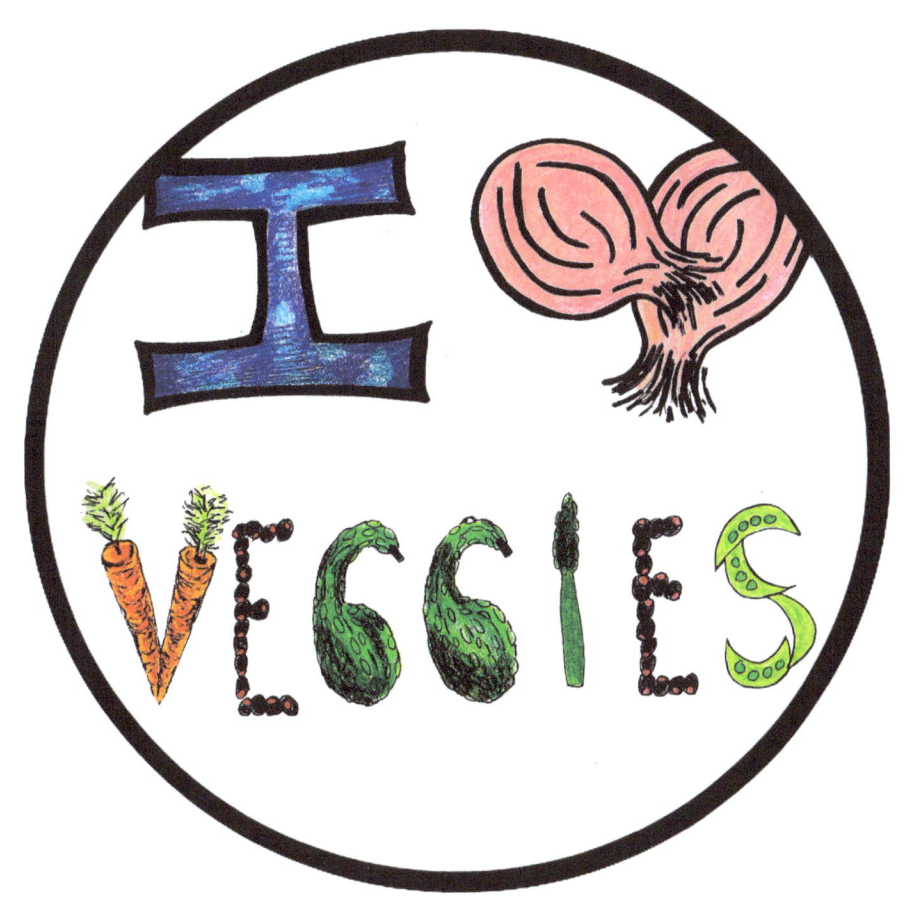

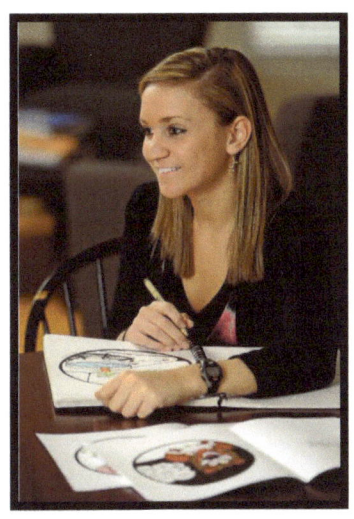

ABOUT THE AUTHOR

Gina Colaizzo is a graduate of Lafayette College with major in Neuroscience and a minor in Art. She also recently received a Bachelor of Science in Nursing from Johns Hopkins University. In combining her interests in science, art and pediatric medicine, she hopes to advocate for pediatric wellness by producing a series of educational children's books that illustrate and promote healthy lifestyles. As she continues to pursue a career to become a pediatric nurse practitioner, *How To Be a Winner for Dinner* is the first of a series of books she plans to write to achieve this goal.